Fitness Over 60 For Women – How to Stay Fit And Healthy As You Age

Dr. Robertino Bedenian

Published by Dr. Robertino Bedenian, 2024.

While every precaution has been taken in the preparation of this book, the publisher assumes no responsibility for errors or omissions, or for damages resulting from the use of the information contained herein.

FITNESS OVER 60 FOR WOMEN – HOW TO STAY FIT AND HEALTHY AS YOU AGE

First edition. January 13, 2024.

Copyright © 2024 Dr. Robertino Bedenian.

ISBN: 979-8224011940

Written by Dr. Robertino Bedenian.

Also by Dr. Robertino Bedenian

Fitness Over 60 For Women – How to Stay Fit And Healthy As You Age

Does Back Pain Go Away? 10 Answers To The Most Acute Back Pain Issues

Massage Bible - A Beginners Guide To Western And Eastern Massage Therapy

Going Vegan - How To Vegan Without Going Crazy

Chiropraktik - Was Steckt Eigentlich Dahinter?

Massagen: Ein Überblick Über Westliche Und Östliche Massagetechniken

Natuerlich Abnehmen, Schlank Und Endlich Fit Sein

P.S. Ich Liebe Dich: Wenn Liebe So Einfach Wäre

Was Tun Bei Rückenschmerzen, Bandscheibenvorfall Und Ischiasschmerzen: 10 Antworten Zu Den Häufigsten Fragen Bei Rückenschmerzen

Was Tun Gegen Schlafapnoe, Schlafstörungen Und Schnarchen

Self-Help Books for Women – How to Overcome Depression, Anxiety, Divorce, Addiction, and Trauma

Diabetes How to Help: Everything You Need to Know About Diabetes Type 1 and Type 2

Diet and Workout Planner: How to Stay Healthy and Get Fit for Life

Everything I Know About Love

The Sleep Easy Solution Book: How to Stop Sleep Apnea, Snoring, and Sleep Disorders

Your Super Gut Feeling Restored – How to Restore Your Life Energy and Overall Health from The Inside Out

Watch for more at https://booksummarypublishing.com.

Table of Contents

Fitness Over 60 for Women

How to Stay Fit and Healthy As You Age

Exercises for Women for Best Way to Get in Shape and Becoming Fit Fast and Easy

Dr. Robertino Bedenian

The author of this book does not dispense medical advice or prescribe the use of any technique as a form of treatment for physical, emotional, or medical problems without the advice of a physician, either directly or indirectly. The intent of the author is only to offer information of a general nature to help you in your quest for emotional, physical, and spiritual well-being. In the event you use any of the information in this book for yourself, the author and the publisher assume no responsibility for your actions.

This book is not intended as a substitute for the medical advice of physicians. The reader should regularly consult a physician in matters relating to his/her health and particularly with respect to any symptoms that may require diagnosis or medical attention.

Please consult a medical or health professional before you begin any exercise, nutrition, or supplementation program or if you have questions about your health.

The information in this book is meant to supplement, not replace, proper training. Like any sport exercises involving equipment, balance and environmental factors, these exercises pose some inherent risk. The author and publisher advise readers to take full responsibility for their safety and know their limits. While practicing the skills described in this book, be sure you do not take risks beyond your level of experience, aptitude, training, and comfort level.

Preface

Maintaining fitness is very important as it helps your muscles grow stronger. Doing regular physical activity can prevent many health problems that come with age. As women age, their bodies undergo many physiological changes. If you are 60 or above this age, then it is the right time to get in shape doing moderate exercises to stay fit and healthy. Physical appearance is not as important as physical health. There are plenty of ways to improve your physical activity such as cycling, walking, sports, active recreation, and playing. Women above 60 must start weekly physical activity. They should start with multi-component physical activity. When you are over 60, stretching is one of the safest and easiest exercises you can do to stay fit. It should never hurt or make you feel bad to exercise. Try doing ten-minute interval exercises twice a day. Static exercises, also known as intermittent exercises, are those in which a body is held at a specific single position and muscles are stretched at high intensities for a certain period without feeling pain and without the movement of the joint. Yoga provides far-fetched benefits for an older population to help them maintain their balance, keep their joints flexible, maintain their bone health and muscle mass, slow down their aging process, and teach them how to cope with their mental state. Nutrition along with physical activity can improve the fitness of women above 60.

CHAPTER 1: Introduction

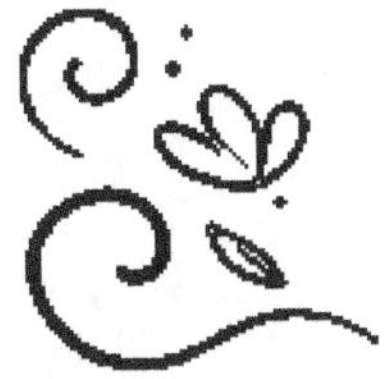

It is essential for older adults especially women to care for themselves. The best way they can take care of themselves is by doing regular physical activity to improve their health and fitness. Doing regular physical activity can prevent many health problems that come with age. Maintaining fitness is very important as it helps your muscles grow stronger. This way, you can easily carry out day-to-day activities without being dependant on anyone. Always make a routine to do regular physical activity. If you cannot do exercises regularly, then at least do it on some days during the week as some physical activity is better than none at all. In the next pages, you will see various health benefits of doing exercise that will in turn make you stronger to do more physical activity. Older women above the age of 60 may have some chronic conditions due to bad dietary habits, lack of exercise and physical activity, or hereditary factors. These women must include exercise in their daily life to combat the diseases and live a longer, healthier life. Many women cannot do physical activity due to these chronic conditions such as arthritis, cardiovascular disease, respiratory diseases, etc. Mostly, women over 60 are not able to do 150 minutes of moderate aerobic activity in a week because of these diseases. They should try to be physically more active according to the pace of their body. Women over the age of 60 tend to have a sedentary lifestyle with little to no exercise and minimal physical activity. These habits can further deteriorate their health condition and fitness. Exercise is essential to stay fit and active throughout their life. By doing the right exercises, women of older age can slow down or even reverse the aging process. Doing exercise regularly helps you stay active and fit. These women often have fewer health issues. Many women specially working women have an active lifestyle until they reach 60. After 60, the physical activity becomes zero as there is not much to do. If you are 60 or above this age, then it is the right time to start exercising again to stay fit and healthy.

Changes in body Over 60

As women age, their bodies undergo many physiological changes. Their skin turns to be more dry than usual. Skin itchiness becomes common. Skin starts to look like a crepe or tissue paper. Dark spots, wrinkles, creases, and bruises are more noticeable after 60. The wounds on the skin take longer to heal. But, there is no need to worry if you have been active throughout your life and tend to be active in the future, too. All these processes can be slowed down by doing regular physical activity. If you have been active during early life and your 60s, your joints, muscles, and bones can stay in pretty good shape. Because of cartilage wear, lack of lubricating joint fluid, and weakened muscles, aging and inactivity can cause achy joints. Maintaining a healthy weight and strength training are two options. Weight-bearing behaviors cause the bones to become stronger and denser, reducing the risk of fractures and osteoporosis. Older women must take Vitamin D and calcium supplementation. The recommended dose of Vitamin D per day for women above 60 is 600 International Units. For women above 70, the range is 800 International Units per day. Calcium requirements for women above 60 are 1200 mg per day.

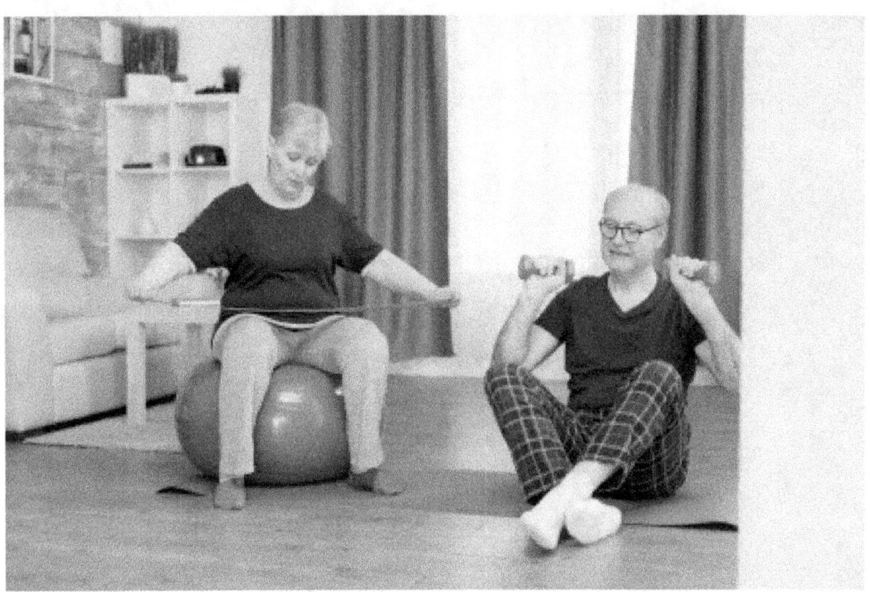

The creaking and popping noises in your joints may sound like breaking twigs, but they're generally not severe unless they're followed by pain and swelling. Even if your metabolism decreases by up to 5% every decade, you don't have to add weight in your 60s. Simply stay healthy and eat fewer calories if necessary. Other issues that arise after age 60 for women may be less production of hydrochloric acid due to which the absorption of Vitamin B12 is hindered. Always consult your doctor to take your Vitamin B12 supplementation. The optimal dose of Vitamin B12 is 2.4 mcg daily for women above 60. This occurs due to the reason that your stomach empties at a slower rate. This increases the chances of reflux. This can also lead to constipation which is a very common problem for women of older age. The best way to get relief from this is to eat more fiber and drink more water throughout the day. The chances of developing colon polyps also decrease when eating more fibrous food. These types of polyps can lead to cancer. Hence, it is very important to eat more fiber daily. Another problem women of older age face is that they get very thirsty due to dehydration. So, it is very important to drink water even if you are not thirsty.

Signs of Aging

Even the most beautiful and brightest stars have to fade one day. Similarly, the most beautiful faces eventually find their bodies drooping and sag or wrinkle as they age. That is the natural aging process and it is inevitable. There are plenty of ways to reduce or slow down the aging process. But first, let us discuss some signs of aging. Physical appearance is not as important as physical health. Keep that in mind! There are many pitfalls of age-related issues such as heart diseases or dementia. These issues come at an early stage if a woman is not physically active in her life. You can be sure that the efforts you put in to achieve fitness are preserved. You will learn plenty of tips and tricks to start moving better, feeling better, and living an active and healthy lifestyle to attain fitness.

Lifestyle Changes for Fitness

Walking for Heart Health: Many women start to feel that their endurance and energy start to decrease after the age of 60. So, in order to avoid this issue, they should make walking a part of their daily routine because walking is an ideal way to add exercise to your life without working too hard. It is less strenuous than running. But to reap the most benefits you must walk for a longer duration. The World Health Organization recommends 30 minutes of regularly walking for 5 days a week.

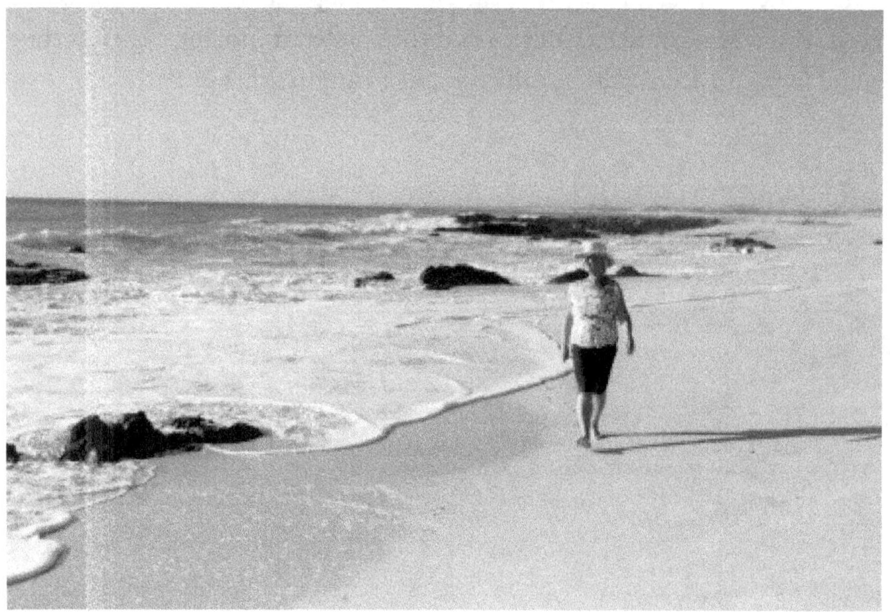

Keep Your Bones Healthy

A very common bone disease that comes up with age is osteoporosis. It causes fragile bones. It affects around 22 million women after the age of 50 in Europe alone. Medications are taken by most women to slow it but there is no permanent cure. To avoid or slow it down, start stair climbing, cross-training machines, moderate weight lifting, brisk walking, gardening, and working out with resistance bands. All these activities will help you reduce the rate of natural bone loss that starts to occur after age 35.

Eat some Brain Food

Eating smart is taught at all ages. Recently, many dementia cases alarmed the doctors and they emphasized eating healthier especially brain foods. Eating healthy foods that protect and nourish your brain cells is very essential for your mind and body's well-being. Brain foods aren't very complex foods. They are simple dietary choices that include eating lots of fish, fruits, vegetables, olive oil, and omega 3 fatty acids. These foods help nourish your grey matter and they provide plenty of energy that is required to stay healthy and fit at the age of 60.

Laugh a Lot

This does not mean that you need to keep on laughing without any cause. Just focus on staying positive. Laugh helps to release the happy hormone such as endorphins which is essential to keep your body fit and healthy. These hormones stop the degenerative changes in the body that occur due to age. Studies show that people who often laugh are expected to live a longer and healthier life. It protects your heart by decreasing the stress hormones, releasing the happy hormones, increasing blood flow, and increasing infection-fighting antibodies in the blood. Just focus on getting those endorphins high by laughing and even joining a dance class. This way, you will boost your energy, increase life expectancy, and improve your fitness.

Stop Smoking and Drinking Alcohol

As you age, your body reacts differently to smoking and alcohol consumption. Around 29 million people have chronic liver diseases due to excessive alcohol consumption. Mostly these chronic diseases show up after the age of 60. Smoking alone can cause lung cancer that will destroy your lungs and your health. Alcoholism is also responsible for bad health and fitness. Even if you drink 1 glass a day and do exercise regularly, your body will not be able to cope up with the damage caused by alcohol. So, stop smoking or drinking alcohol if you want to stay fit after 60. You will see many positive changes in your body once you stop smoking. All these guidelines are very important if you want to maintain your health after 60.

CHAPTER 2: Physical Activity

What is Physical Activity?

The definition of physical activity given by the World Health Organization (WHO) is any bodily movement that is produced by skeletal muscles. It requires energy expenditure. It means all movements that are done in leisure time, moving from one place to another or a part of work. Health is improved by both moderate and vigorous physical activity.

There are plenty of ways to improve your physical activity such as cycling, walking, sports, active recreation, and playing. You can also have joy while doing regular physical activity.

Women aged 60 years and above

Women above age 60 must start weekly physical activity. They should start with multi-component physical activity. This will improve the functional balance. They should also do strength training at moderate or greater intensity 3 days per week. This will enhance functional capacity and prevent age-related falls.

In adults and older adults, higher levels of physical activity impede:

- risk of death from any cause
- risk of death from cardiovascular disease
- occurrence of hypertension
- occurrence of site-specific cancers (bladder, breast, colon, endometrial, esophageal adenocarcinoma, gastric, and renal cancers)
- occurrence of type-2 diabetes
- mental wellbeing (reduced anxiety and depression symptoms)
- cognitive health
- sleep
- adiposity measurements are improved

There are certain policies for safe physical activity. Physical activity policies seek to ensure that:

- walking, cycling, and other active non-motorized ways of movement are available and safe for everyone.
- labor and workplace policies promote active commuting and opportunities for becoming physically active during the workday
- childcare, schools, and higher education institutions provide supportive and safe spaces and facilities for all students to spend their free time actively
- community-based and school-sport programs offer equal opportunities for all ages and abilities.
- primary and secondary schools provide quality physical education that assists children in developing behavior habits that will keep them physically involved throughout their lives.

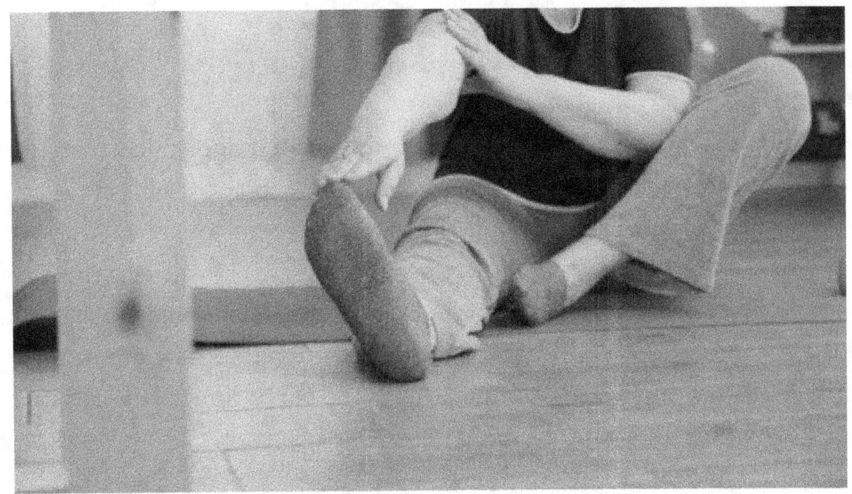

- health care services advise and help patients to be physically active on a daily basis.
- sports and fitness centers offer opportunities for all to access and engage in a range of sports, dance, exercise, and active recreation.

Here are some exercises that will help women above 60 to get in shape.

Stretching Out

When you're over 60, stretching is one of the safest and easiest exercises you can do to stay fit. Raise your arm as high as you can for stretching exercises, and repeat the process with your other arm. Keep them for a total of 5 seconds. It should be done three times. There is another way to do stretching. Stand up and hold a chair with your left hand. After that raise your right knee and hold that foot with your right hand. Now bring the heel to the ground. Hold it for 5 seconds and then release. Repeat this step three times. You can do the same exercise while you sit on the floor (see the image below).

Standing on One Leg

Balancing and standing is a very easy exercise for women above 60. It is a complex exercise that involves many muscle groups such as the inner ears, eyes, and receptors in the joints. By balancing regularly, you will restore these muscles' strength. If you want to perform this exercise, then raise your toes and then drop them. Repeat it 10 to 20 times. Now sit and stand up from the chair without the support of your hands. Do these steps 10 to 20 times.

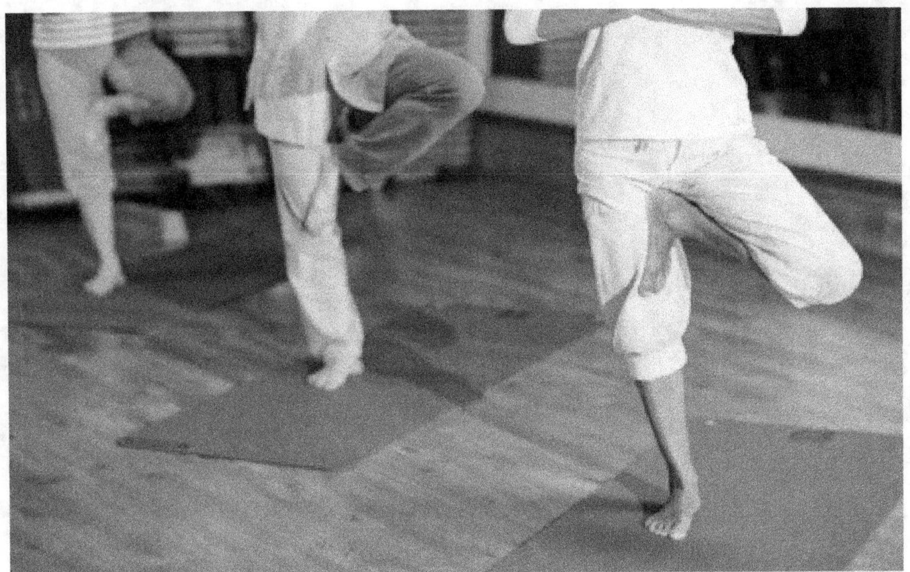

Walk Everyday

After 60, women typically don't walk. It is recommended to walk for at least 25 minutes daily. This will enhance your lifespan by almost 7 years. It will also help repair your DNA in the cells. Start with 15 minutes of walking for 6 days a week in order to stay healthy and fit. You can also climb stairs 5-10 times a day or do jogging for 10 minutes a day.

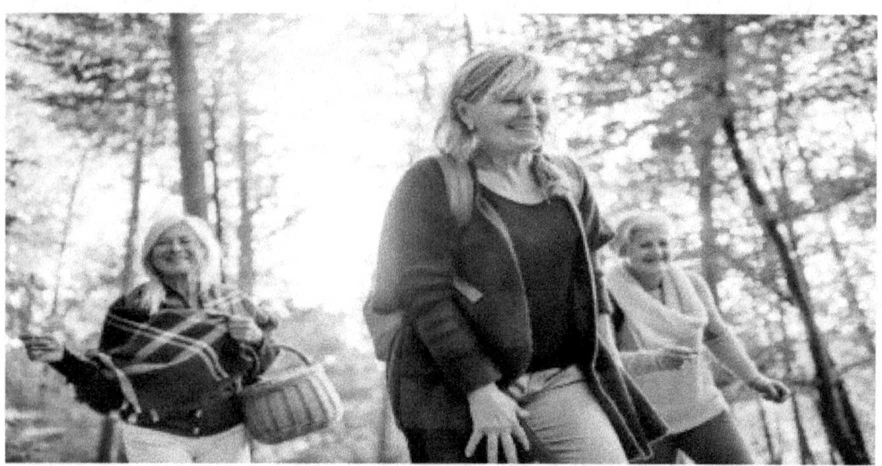

Breathing During Exercises

Each relaxed breath moves about 0.5 liters of air into the lungs of the average person. During intense exercise, this amount will rise to 3 liters.

While doing strength training, the gold standard is to inhale during relaxation and exhale during exertion. When doing cardio, you usually breathe in and out through your nose or, as the pressure increases, through your mouth.

Here are a few breathing techniques to use while doing exercise:

- Encourage yourself to hold the breath to count out loud each repetition.
- Exhale during the left footfall (not the right) if you are experiencing side-stitches when running.
- If you are having trouble breathing, then stand up with your hands behind the head to open the lungs to allow for deeper inhalation.
- Use the talk test to determine the intensity of the exercise. If you can't talk much, you are in the high-intensity zone. The intensity is low to moderate if you still can have a conversation. Deep, steady breathing helps relax the body and assists in healing while calming down or stretching.

Breathing through the top of the chest is more normal than breathing deeply through the abdomen using the diaphragm. When you breathe through your chest, you use a lot of ancillary muscles, like those in your neck, that you don't need to use. This can also reinforce neck and shoulder pain, which is common among women over 60.

Breathing smoothly and rhythmically, regardless of the pattern, will help athletes relax. It's difficult to get into the zone if your breathing is irregular if you're busting out your last track interval, or burning through your last set of squats.

CHAPTER 3: Exercises for Beginners

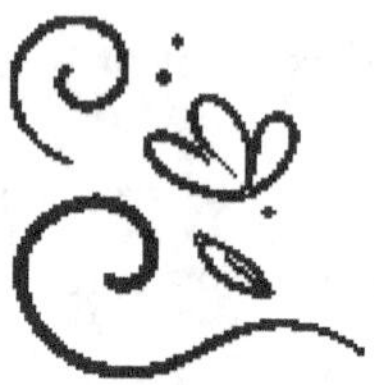

It should never hurt or make you feel bad to exercise. If you feel dizzy or out of breath, develop chest pain or pressure, break out in a cold sweat, or experience pain, stop exercising immediately and call your doctor. If a joint is red, swollen, or algesic, stop doing what you're doing—the easiest way to deal with injuries is to prevent them in the first place. If you have pain or discomfort after exercising, consider exercising for shorter periods but more often during the day.

Start slow and build up steadily. If you haven't been active for a while, start slowly and work your way up. Try doing ten-minute interval exercises twice a day. Alternatively, try only one class per week. If you're worried about falling or have a heart condition, start with simple chair exercises to gradually improve your fitness and confidence.

Prevent injury and discomfort by warming up, cooling down, and keeping water handy. Commit to an exercise routine for at least three or four weeks so it becomes a habit, and then push yourself to stick to it. This is much easier if you find things that you enjoy.

Pilates

For enhancing rehabilitation in the physical therapist community, Pilates was introduced. Pilate's technique can be used to enhance muscle strength, stability, range of motion, flexibility, and proprioception. It is very much efficient for functional movement patterns. Movement requires both physical control and mental focus. There are different types of Pilates: you can perform exercises on the floor, workout mats, or sitting on a Swiss ball while trying to keep the balance.

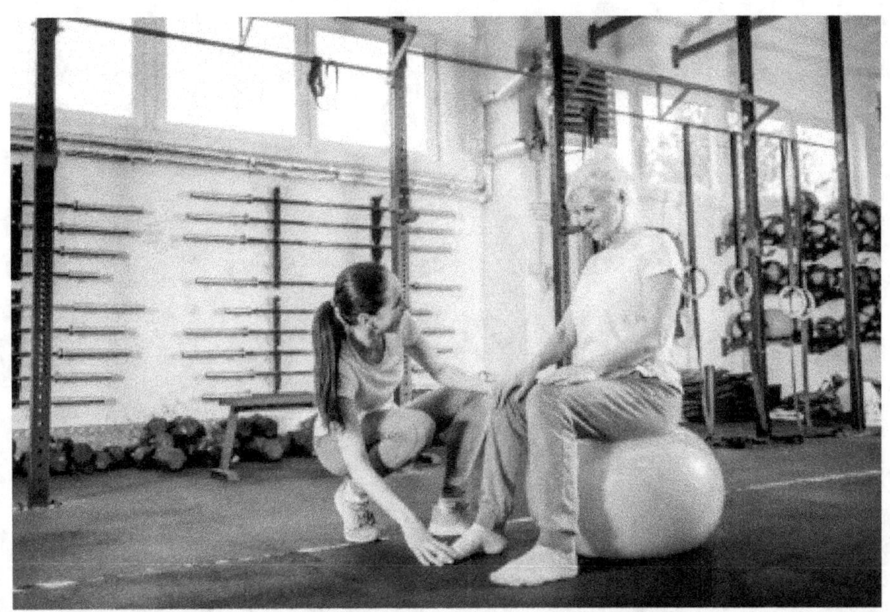

If you want to do Pilates, there are different types of Pilates but for elderly women spine Pilates is more effective. Get yourself dressed, bring a yoga mat, and find a flat surface area to lie on. Do exhale inhale properly. Squeeze and lift your hips into the air until your body forms a straight line between your shoulders and the head. Then press your weight equally into your feet, shoulders, and limbs. Exhale or inhale three times while holding a pose. Adjust to the floor by lowering yourself (see the image below).

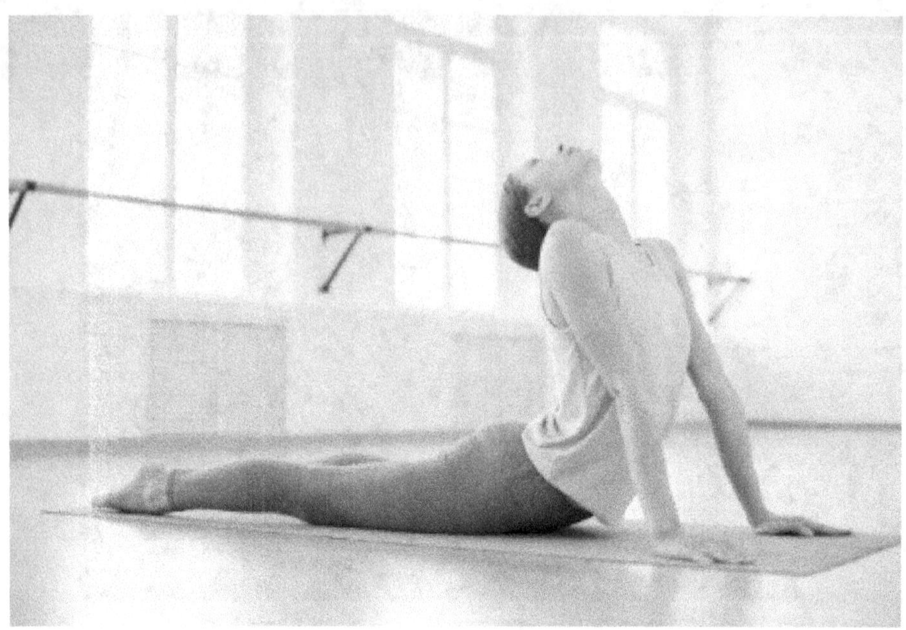

Tai chi

Tai chi is one of the ancient Chinese exercises also known as" meditation in motion". It is a combination of slow and relaxed movements involving the brain, body, and soul. For promoting balance, flexibility, and cardiovascular disease with older patients tai chi appears to be safe. Tai chi helps in pain reduction, blood pressure reduction, stress reduction, improved sleep patterns and increases the quality of life.

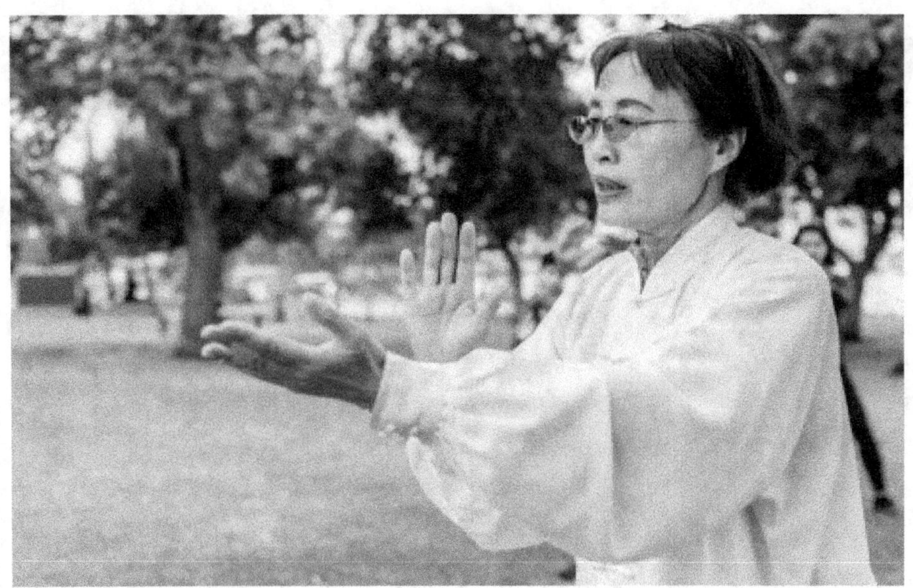

Swimming

Swimming is a low-impact, non-weight-bearing activity. It imposes no strain on the spine, knees, or hips. In addition, the buoyancy of water maintains some of the body weight and decreases the force of gravity, trying to relieve some of the regular strain on these joints. Swimming activates all major muscle groups resulting in stronger muscles, especially the upper body, core muscles, and leg muscles (all essential muscle groups for posture and stabilization) which reduces the chance of falling. Senior women should try swimming 3 times a week for optimum health and quality.

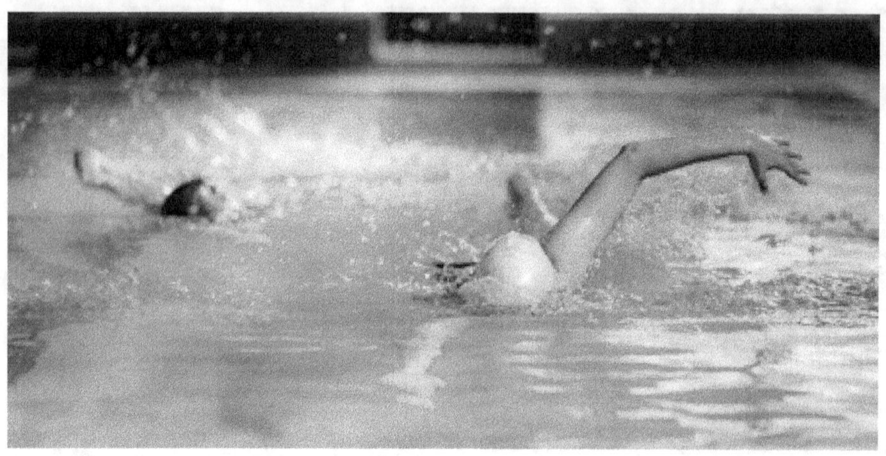

Jogging

Jogging or running helps burning calories, preventing the risk of Osteoarthritis by maintaining weight. Jogging helps maintain cardiovascular health. When you run blood flows through the lungs, which dramatically increases the oxygenated blood. By doing jogging regularly, you will avoid diseases like breast, colon, and lung cancer. You will also stay far from stroke and diabetes. If you're new to exercising or out of shape, start by walking to give your body time to adjust. Walk for 15-30 minutes a day 3-4 days a week, and gradually increase your walking speed to jogging.

Stretching

Lunges help you increase core strength, strengthen your lower body and muscle tissues. It also helps in maintaining weight by burning calories. This can help in achieving your proper balance and coordination. In lunges, flexor muscles are highly focused which brings flexibility to the body. Lunges help in removing extra strain on your spine while working on other parts of the body. Stand straight, keeping your body straight, lift your chin and relax your shoulders. Establish one leg forward when lowering the hips so both knees are bent at a 90-degree angle. Make sure your knees are in line with your ankles. Make certain that the other knee must not come in contact with the ground. Maintain your body weight on your heels. Now switch feet and do the same thing again. Do it 10 times for one leg with 3 sets of repetitions.

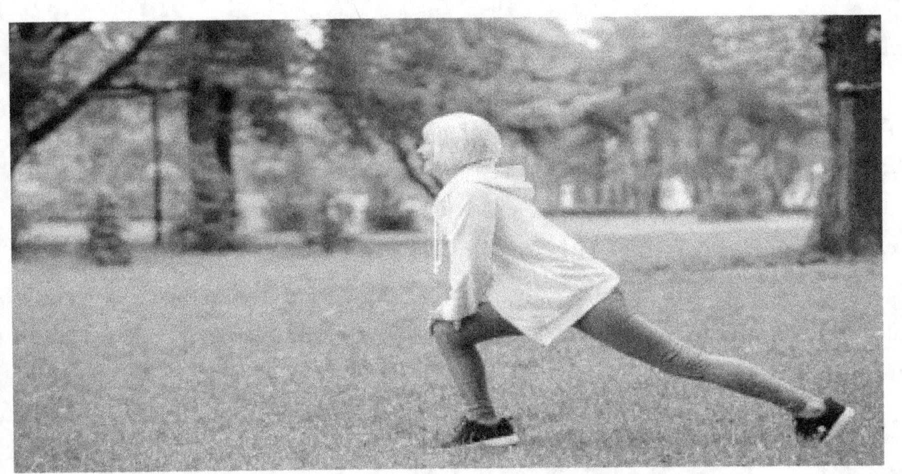

Cycling

During cycling, body muscles move in a smooth motion that doesn't put any extra stress on the body. Weight gain is a major problem in elder people because they become inactive. Cycling is a good way to stay active and burn calories. The combination of cycling with low-impact exercise like swimming helps to maintain weight as you age. Cycling is recommended for seniors especially because of their memory gap, dementia, and Alzheimer's disease. During cycling your body works at maximum capacity, ensuring that the brain is fully oxygenated. Do at least 30 to 45 minutes of cycling daily.

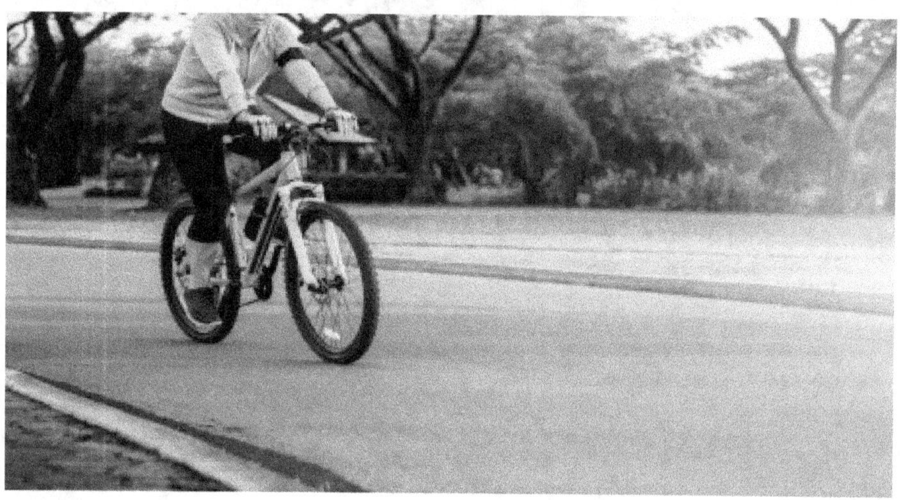

Mini Squats

Mini squats help strengthen knee muscles and cartilage involving the knee joint. Squats also help support weight-bearing joints (knee, hips, ankle) by making them stronger. If you want to feel more secure doing this exercise due to balance issues, place your hands on the back of the chair and stand with your feet hip-width apart. Slowly bend your knees as much as you can while having them facing forward. Make sure that your knees don't bend over your big toe. Retain a straight back at all times. Bring yourself back up to a standing position slowly, squeezing (clenching) your buttocks as you need it. Repeat it 5 times.

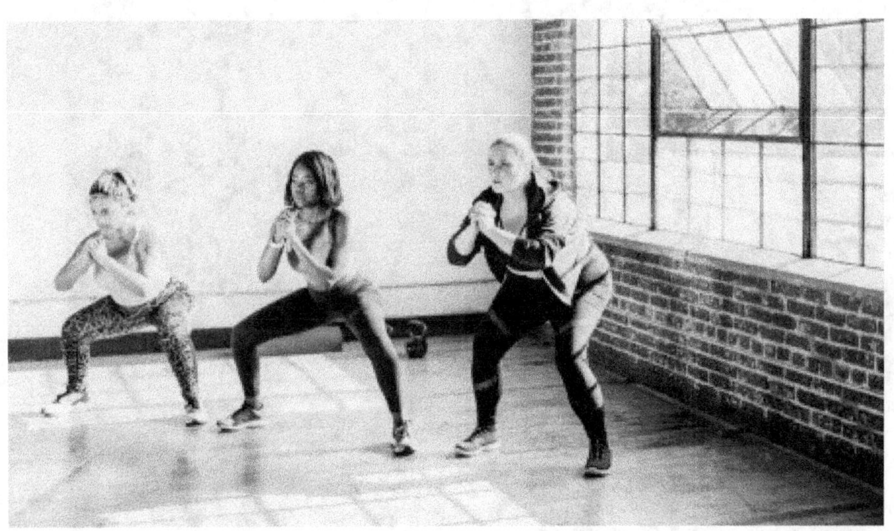

Bridge

Major problems of seniors are linked to lower back issues which are one of the causes of immobility as you age. Bridges are highly effective for strengthening glutes muscles. It activates all core muscles including transverse abdominous, rectus abdominous, and obliques which helps the body to do better functions by improving posture. Lay on your back with your hands at your sides and your feet about 10 inches from your buttocks tightly flat on the floor. Hold your pelvis in the air for 30 seconds, thrusting it as hard as you can. Repeat it 3-4 times.

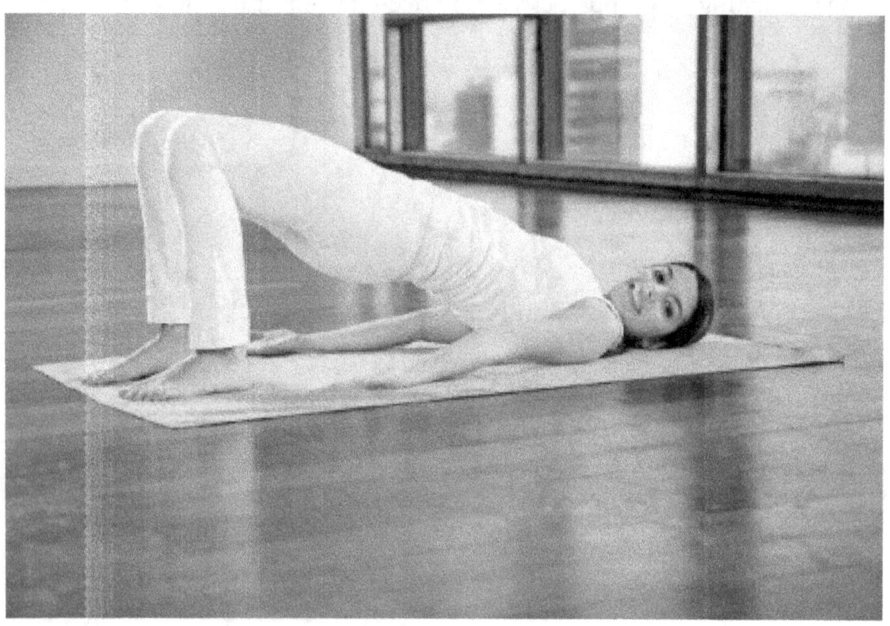

Plank

Plank helps strengthen both your deep core muscles and abdominals which are not easy muscles to target during the workout. By doing plank you can develop or maintain these muscles. This also helps you improve your posture and reduces back pain. Lie down with your stomach flat on the floor. Then lift your body straight up by placing your elbows on the ground. Make sure that your knees don't touch the floor while keeping the rest of your body upright, facing down toward the floor. Keep a plank position with your body for 30 seconds to a minute. If you can make it 30 seconds in this position, you can scale this exercise by placing only your hands (not the elbows) on the floor while lifting your body up and keeping it straight in this position for 30 seconds (see the image below).

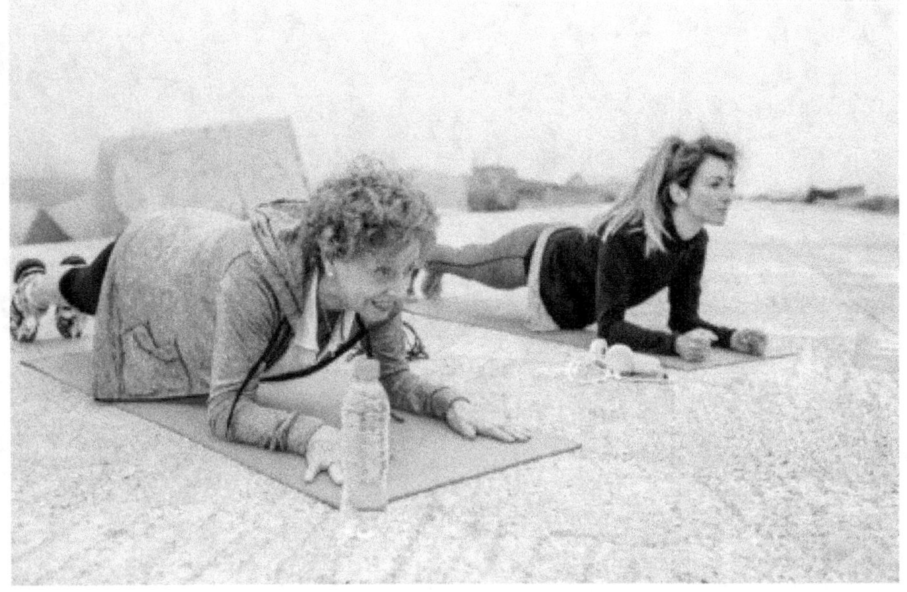

Leg Raises

Leg lifts tend to strengthen the lower abs, butt, and hip flexors, all of which contribute to balance and mobility. Place your hands under your lower back for stability when lying on your back. Lift one leg slowly 6-10 inches off the ground and hang for 30 seconds. Repeat 10 times for each leg.

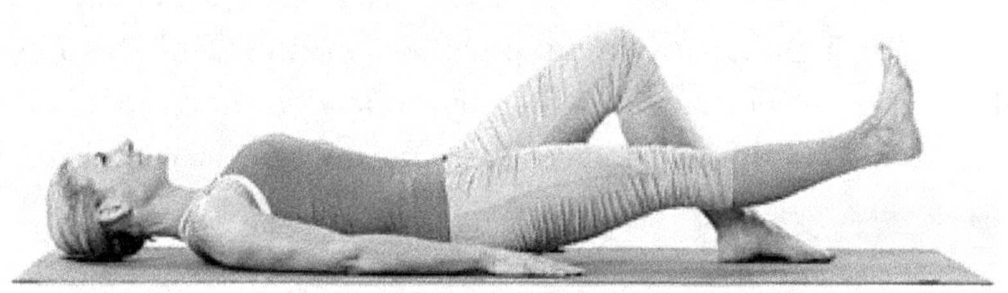

CHAPTER 4: Static Exercises

Our body is like a car, in which the engine not only needs gas but it is important to use it as well. If we park our car in a garage and do not use it for a longer time, it will cause trouble after some time and the battery will run out of charge although there is still enough gas in the engine. Similarly, our bodies not only need food but also physical exercise as they both work synergistically. If we just eat and eat and do not make our muscles active, our body will be just like a dead battery of a car. Food and exercise together keep our body healthy as exercise is crucial for your body. But the main question is which specific type of exercises are beneficial for you, specifically for your physical condition as you age? Two major types of exercises are commonly discussed; dynamic and static exercises. In this chapter, we will distinctively discuss static exercises, how you can benefit from them, and most importantly, how women over 60 can benefit from static exercises.

Static exercises

Static exercises, also known as intermittent exercises, are those in which a body is held at a specific single position and muscles are stretched at high intensities for a certain period without feeling pain, without the movement of the joint. Usually, the body is held in a position for up to 45 seconds with 2-3 times repetitions. No matter how old we, we need a flexible body. Flexibility becomes even more crucial as we age. So, for elderly people, flexibility is a necessity. We can say, being flexible is one of the critical components for a good health and fitness level.

Dynamic Exercises

Apart from this, we should know about dynamic exercises as well. Contrary to static stretching, dynamic stretching involves movement. These exercises are done, along with warm-up, at the beginning of a workout. After all, it prepares your muscles and other tissues and ligaments to perform well and function effectively for exercises whereas static stretching is done at the end of the workout because you have already warmed your body up. It takes the body to the resting phase and slows down muscles after exercise.

List of Static Exercises

If you are a fitness freak, it's not enough to know only about what static exercises are. If you're eager to know which types of exercises are involved in static exercises, this chapter will surely help you. Here is the list of some static stretching that you can adopt for your exercise routine. Posterior capsule stretch

1. Hamstring stretch
2. Quadriceps stretch
3. Biceps stretch
4. Chest stretch
5. Upper back stretch
6. Shoulder stretch
7. Shoulder and triceps stretch
8. Side bends
9. Hip and thigh stretch
10. Front of trunk stretch
11. Calf stretch
12. Abdominal and lower back muscles stretch

In the next subchapter (The Senior's stretching plan), we will cover static exercises specially tailored for seniors that are performed by a professional female fitness instructor. Watch the video below carefully so you know exactly how to do these exercises properly.

Benefits of Static Exercises

Now we'll enlighten some of the beneficial effects of static exercises.

- **Enhanced Range of Motion**

Range of motion is defined by what extent a joint of a body can move comfortably in a particular direction. Static stretching is important to improve the range of motion of joints at the end of your exercise or workout. It makes the body perform daily routine tasks easily and with comfort. It increases the tolerance level of a person to stretch the muscles and joints. Range of motion is positively affected as these stretches make the joint combat more stretching force. Muscle length or extensibility is not increased in static exercises.

- **Injury prevention**

Another important benefit of static exercise is quite fascinating. Apart from making your body stretchable and flexible, these exercises are beneficial in preventing the body from injuries. If your muscles are overstretched and tight from extraneous exercises, static stretching is an effective way to decrease the stiffness of your muscles and joints and helps in reducing pain. One of the research depicts that static stretches decrease the risk of bodily injuries which are caused during different sports and exercises like strain injuries and sprain injuries.

- **Improves Blood Circulation**

If we make our muscles stronger by static exercises, it will increase the blood flow of the body and make our blood circulation effective, thus positively affecting our body.

- **Flexibility**

Women over 60 profit from static stretching as it makes the body flexible enough to make their body easier to move by improving muscle strength, improving their speed and agility. Not only athletes, dancers, and people doing gymnastics can make their body stretch tolerant by using these exercises in their daily routine. Research studies showed that static stretching improves sprinting time if exercise is done three times weekly for a total of 6 weeks. For women interested in different sports and who want to make their body active, these exercises, if done for a shorter duration, can be an essential warm-up component. It will make their body more extensible and prevent them from sports injuries.

- **Helping hand for Patients**

If we take a look at the patients facing bone disorders, these exercises can be fruitful for them. Osteoarthritis which damages any joint in your body affects the quality of life negatively. Static Stretching can benefit these patients by improving the range of motion of affected joints. For patients suffering from musculoskeletal pain, including static exercises in their daily routine increases their tolerance level to stretch muscles and joints.

Benefits of Static Exercises for Women above 60 Years of Age

Now, the question is, is there any kind of health or physical benefits that can be obtained by doing static exercises especially for women who are above 60 years of age? The simplest answer is YES. If we go deep, you will be amazed to see how much beneficial it is for women over 60 years. Adults over 65 years must start static stretching if they have been following any exercise regimen.

- **Continue reading to get a quick overview:**

One of the biggest problems with elderly adults is usually limited movement and restricted flexibility. But, this problem can easily be solved with static exercise. It brings a greater level of flexibility along with an increasing range of motion More flexibility means more stretchiness that will probably lead to decreased pain and less stiffness. It will help the person move easily. You would be shocked to know that only a 1-minute hold of static stretches can help achieve superior enhancements in hamstring suppleness with elderly adults. Older adults have to keep the blood flow normally and practicing statics postures can help increase blood flow. It goes without saying but most older adults have spinal issues. By doing only 10 weeks of static stretching, you can see a significant increase in spinal mobility. It means even if the adult has paralysis, it will help him or her recover faster. Static stretching supports normal gait with elderly adults. To maintain a stable walk, try stretching hip flexors and extensors. Ultimately, all the good effects cause older women to function in life properly and efficiently.

The Seniors' Stretching Plan

You are mistaken if you think that stretching after only a couple of days will already help you get the results you want because it demands patience and consistency. Before delving into any stretching program, you need to have the necessary knowledge about how long it is safe to hold stretches for older adults, how often you need stretching, how the static exercises are performed correctly, and what things you might need to avoid when stretching to keep yourself safe from getting an injury.

The Best Stretches for Seniors

For neck:

Neck flexion stretch - 30-60 seconds

Neck extension stretch - 30-60 seconds

Neck side flexion stretch - 30-60 seconds

Neck rotation stretch - 30-60 seconds

Go to

https://for-ever-fit.net/fitness-for-women-over-60-static-exercises-for-neck

to watch the following video for the best **neck** stretches for seniors:

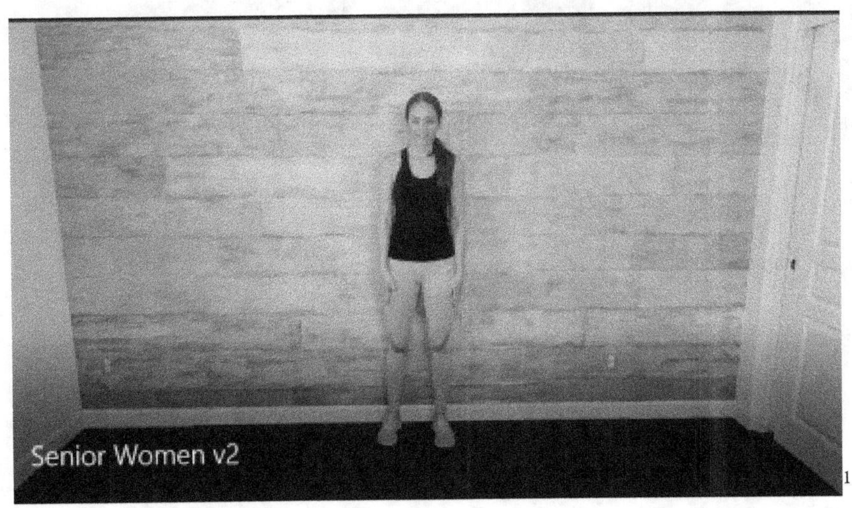

For arms and shoulder:

Levator scapulae stretch - 30-60 seconds

Upper arm & shoulder stretch - 30-60 seconds

Shoulder & arm overhead stretch - 30-60 seconds

---

1. https://www.for-ever-fit.net/fitness-for-women-over-60-static-exercises-for-neck/

Go to

https://for-ever-fit.net/fitness-for-women-over-60-static-exercises-for-arms-and-shoulders

to watch the following video for the best exercises for **arms and shoulders** for seniors:

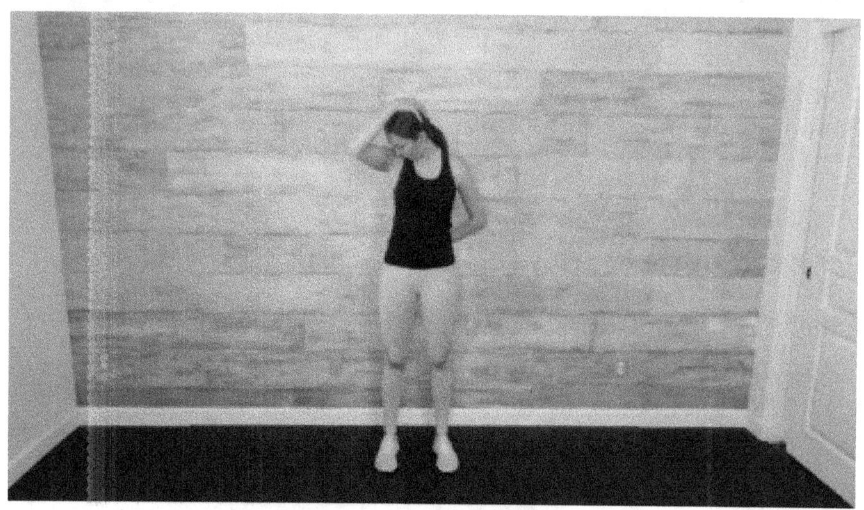

For wrist:

Wrist flexion (forearm) stretch - 30-60 seconds

Wrist extension (forearm) stretch - 30-60 seconds

Go to

https://for-ever-fit.net/static-exercises-for-wrist

to watch the following video for the best **wrist** stretches for seniors:

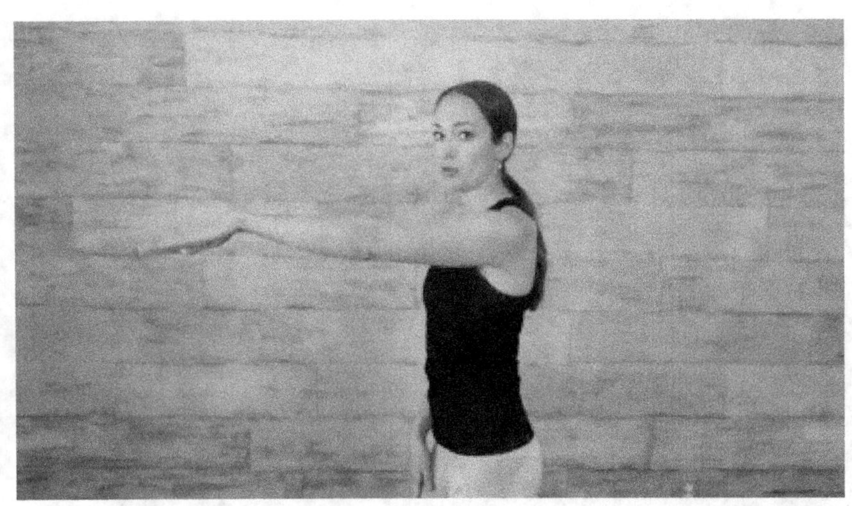

For lumbar:

Lumbar flexion stretches (seated toe touch) - 30-60 seconds

Lumbar side flexion stretches - 30-60 seconds

Lumbar extension stretches - 30-60 seconds

Rhomboids (upper back) stretch - 30-60 seconds

Go to

https://for-ever-fit.net/fitness-for-women-over-60-static-exercises-for-lumbar

to watch the following video for the best **lumbar** stretches for seniors:

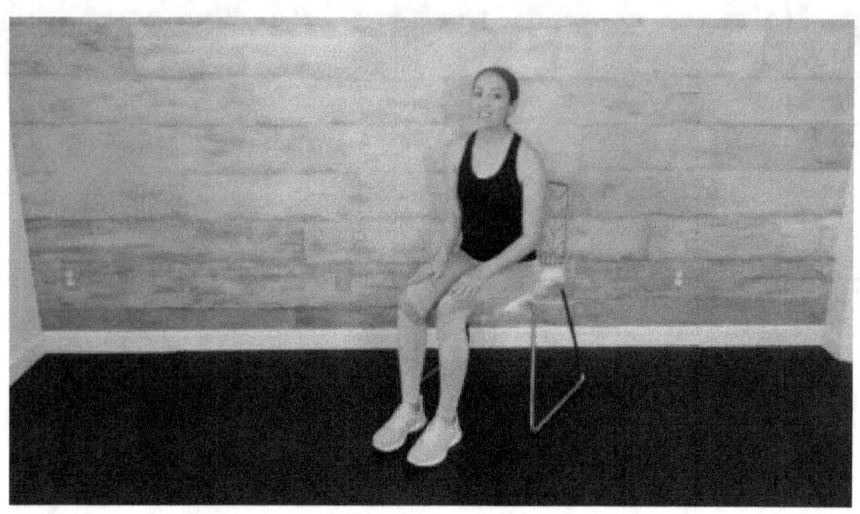

For thoracic region:

Thoracic extension (upper back) stretch - 30-60 seconds

Thoracic rotation (upper back) stretch - 30-60 seconds

For lower body (legs, hamstrings, glutes, thighs, buttocks):

Seated hamstring (back of thigh) stretch - 30-60 seconds

Seated groin (hip adductor) stretch - 30-60 seconds

Seated lateral rotation (hips, buttocks) stretch - 30-60 seconds

Hip flexion (buttocks) stretch - 30-60 seconds

Standing quadriceps (front of thigh) stretch - 30-60 seconds

Standing calf (back of lower leg) stretch - 30-60 seconds

Go to

https://for-ever-fit.net/fitness-for-women-over-60-static-exercises-for-thoracic-extensions

to watch the following video for the best **thoracic** stretches for seniors:

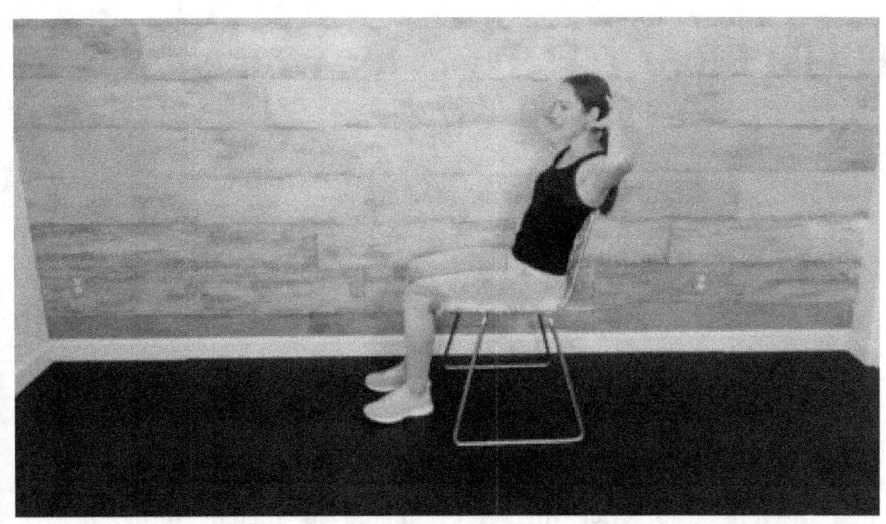

Takeaway points

Stretching is not for only athletes but for everyone.

Always try stretching more than just your muscles and tendons.

Be careful as even a slightly extensive stretching of a tendon (4%) beyond its original length can lead to permanent damage so always warm up first. Never skip stretching after completing running.

CHAPTER 5: Yoga Poses for Women Above 60 Years

Yoga is a disciplined practice that is originated in ancient India. It is a combination of physical, mental, and spiritual exercise or activities. Yoga is one of the six traditional views and schools of Hinduism. It's been around the world for more than 5000 years. It was mainly originated from the Indus Valley civilization and tribal religions of India. After few years, yoga gurus from India introduced these spiritual practices in the West. In India, yoga practices have a meditative as well as spiritual basis while in the west, it was mainly developed into posture-based physical fitness and stress-relief or relaxation technique which helped people to calm down themselves and to take relief from a stressful routine. The word yoga is derived from "Yuj" which is a Sanskrit root that means "to attach or to join". So, the main aim of this Sanskrit-derived word is to join a connection or to form a unity between the "Human Spirit" with a "Divine (Supreme Soul, Lord) Spirit". The main goal of yoga is to attain a state of a brightly shining mind which refers between a purely mental state and a mindful state. But in the Western World, a 3,000 years old tradition yoga is now contemplated as a holistic technique to health and fitness and according to the National Institute of Health it is now also classified as a type of Complementary and Alternative Medicine (CAM)

Yoga Poses for Women Over 60

Yoga provides far-fetched benefits for an older population to help them maintain their balance, keep their joints flexible, maintain their bone health and muscle mass, slows down their aging process as well as teach them how to cope with their mental state. Following are some of the yoga poses that can be easily adapted by seniors and women above 60 years of age to improve focus, concentration, and emotional well-being and to keep their bodies strong and youthful.

- **Mountain Pose**

Mountain Pose is also called the Standing Pose. It looks like the individual is just standing. In this pose, stand tall with big toes touching the base and put the heels slightly apart. Firm your thigh muscles and draw your abdominals in and up and relax your shoulders down and back. Breathe 5 to 8 times while focusing on leg muscles and then slowly release your body. It helps to improve posture, balance, and calm focus. It also strengthens thighs and knees and provides firmness to the abdomen and buttocks.

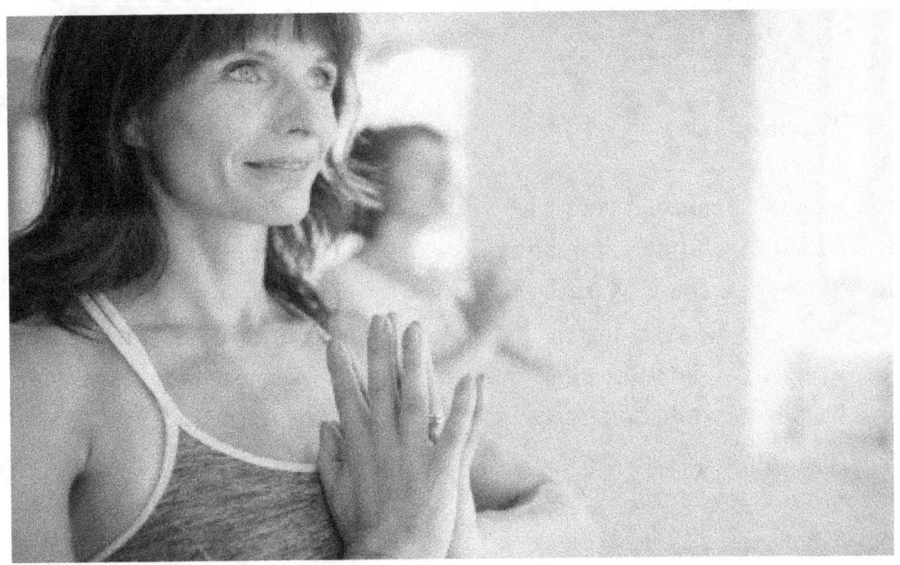

- **Tree Pose**

In this pose, shift your weight into your right foot while lifting your left foot off the floor. Keep your right leg straight and bend your left knee and bring the sole of your left foot towards your inner right thigh. Press your foot into your thigh. Take 6 to 10 breaths, then lower your left foot slowly towards the floor and repeat the same for the other side. This Tree Pose helps to strengthen your legs and core while stretching your inner thighs and groin muscles.

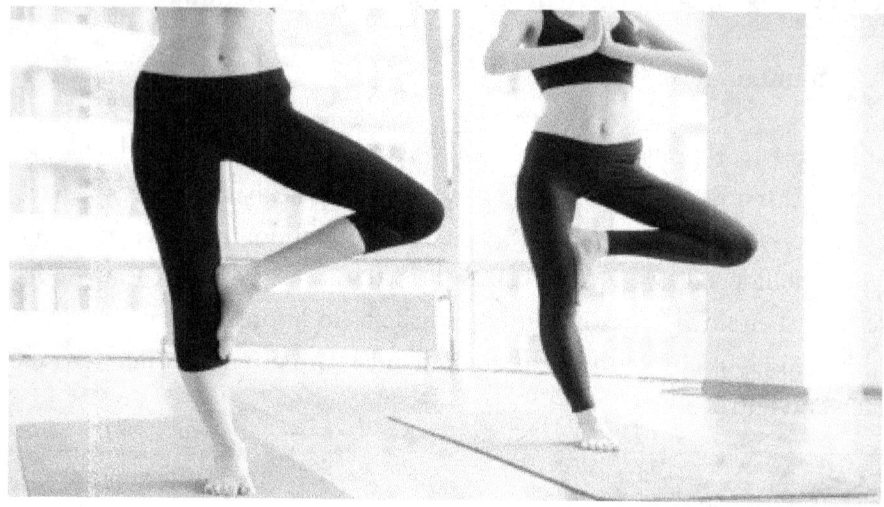

- **Warrior Pose**

This pose helps strengthen your hips and legs and provides better circulation, better respiration, and better stability. Keep your left foot toward the back of your base to come into the Warrior pose. Bring the left heel to the floor and place the toes out at about a 45-degree angle. Then, bend your right knee at about a 90-degree angle. While inhaling, bring your arms up over your head. There is a tenuous backbend while doing this pose that opens the heart and your gaze is towards your fingertips.

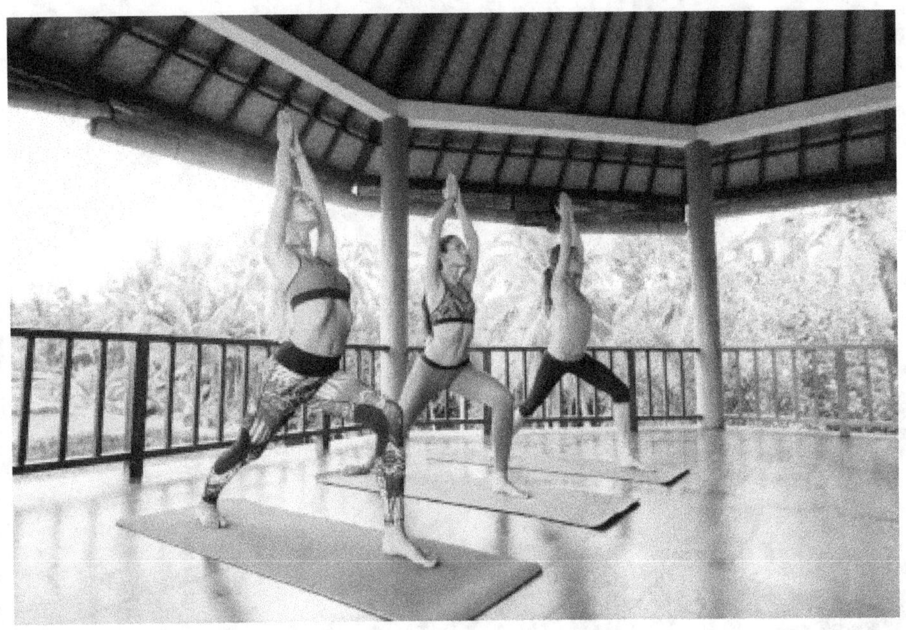

- **Sphinx**

This pose aids in strengthening your upper back and prevents the risk of the forward head syndrome. It gives a firm posture to your upper back portion while strengthening the muscles.

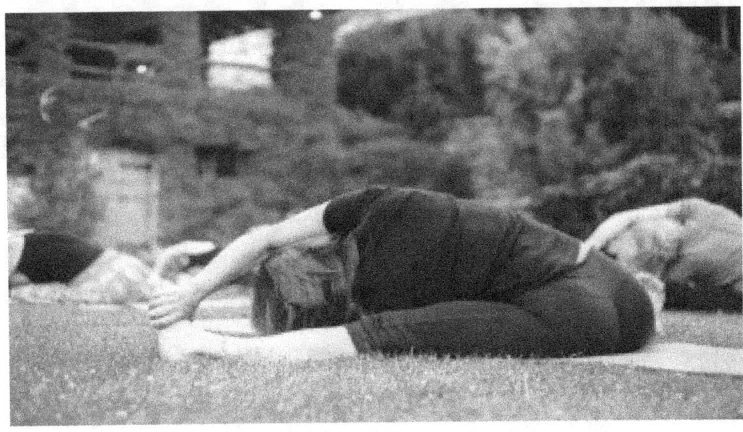

In this pose, you should sit down and bend your shoulders and elbows over your leg. After that, bring the shoulders back away from your neck and feel a tenuous lift in the breast bones. Take 4-7 breaths towards your lower back and abdomen in this pose and then return back to a sitting position.

- **Child Pose**

This pose helps prevent the tension in the shoulders, chest, and back. It also reduces the risks of anxiety and stress and helps ease fatigue. It also aids in better digestion and prevents constipation.

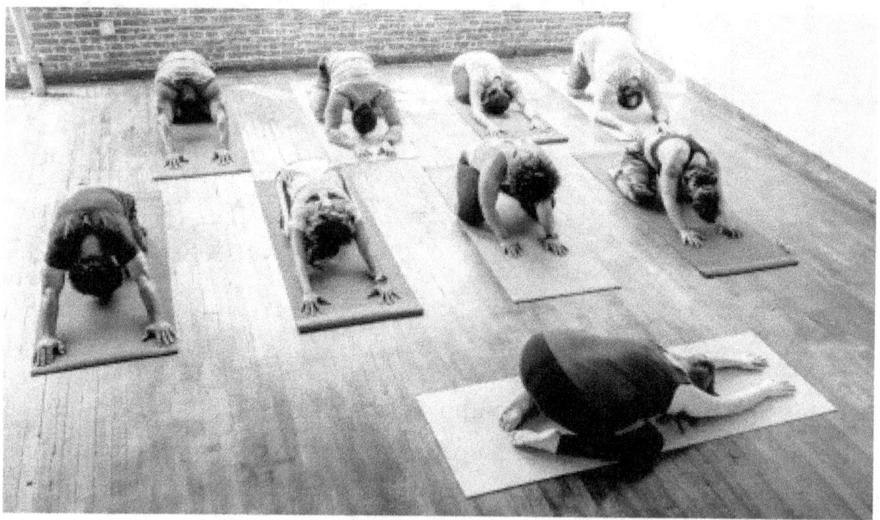

For this pose, you should sit on your heels while keeping your hips on the heels. Bend towards the floor, and lower your forehead to the floor. Keep your arms alongside your body in such a way that hands are on the floor and palms are facing towards the floor. After that, gently press your chest on the thighs. Hold this pose for a few seconds and then slowly come up to sit on the heels.

- **Cobbler's Pose**

This pose is highly effective for seniors as it supports opening up their hips and groins, opens up sciatica, and prevents lower back pain. Moreover, in this pose, they can also massage their feet. For this pose, you should sit tall and bring the soles of your feet together while opening your knees out to the sides. Fold the feet forward for a stretch but try to prevent rounding too much in the lower back. Maintain this position for 6 to 8 breaths and then slowly release this pose.

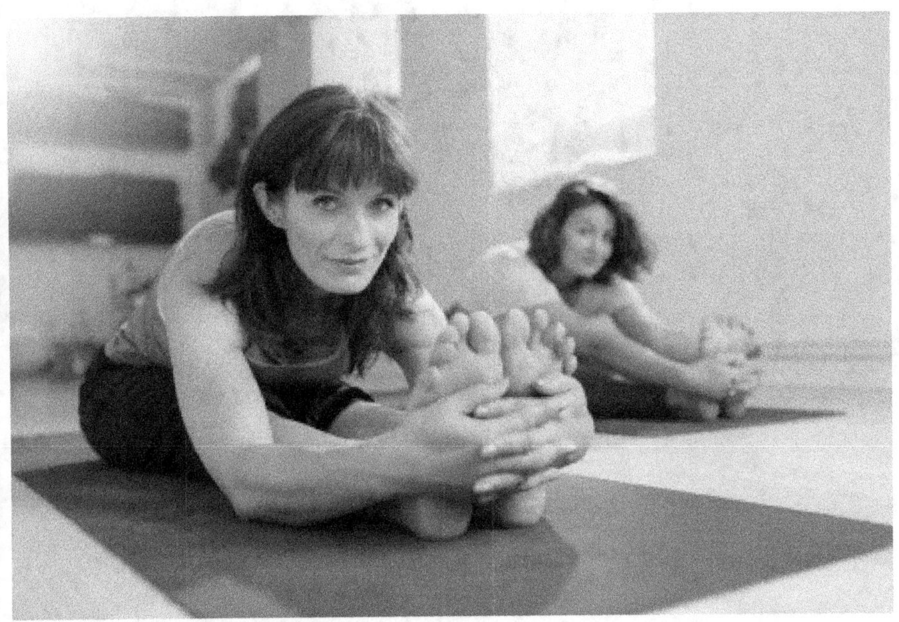

- **Corpse Pose**

This pose should be your last pose while winding out your yoga exercises. It's a perfect example of a relaxation pose in which you relax your body and attain back your energy while focusing on your body and its breathing patterns. This pose resets your nervous system while calming your mind and easing its tension and it also awakens the creativity within the individual and you become more focused on your body and health. In this pose, you just lie down straight on the floor and focus on relaxation and comfort your body.

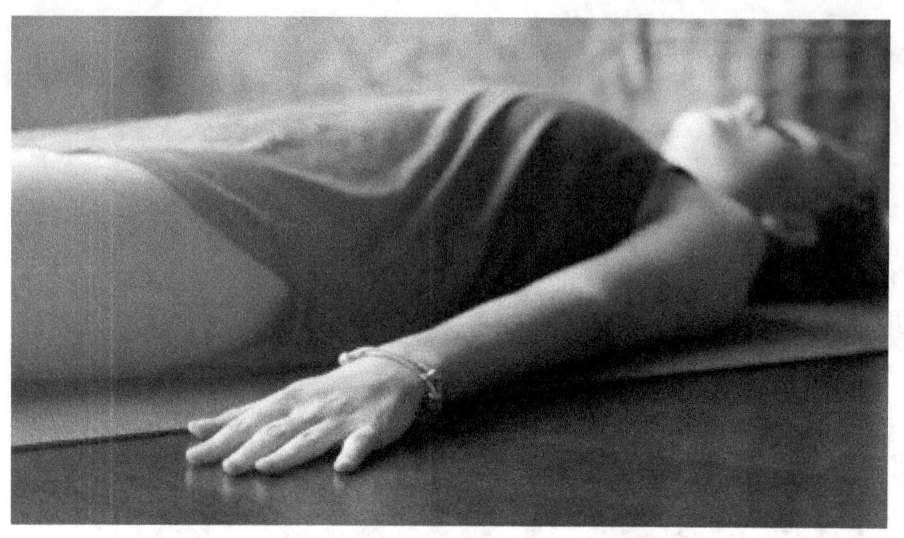

Benefits of Yoga

Yoga is an ancient activity that is designed to bring stability and robustness to the physical, mental, emotional, and spiritual dimensions of the individual.

Following are some of the main benefits of practicing yoga daily:

Regular practice of yoga increases muscle strength, endurance, and flexibility in the human body.

When proper stretching is not done regularly, then muscle fibers cramp which contributes to a bulgy-looking appearance. When an individual does yoga on a regular basis, it increases muscle endurance because this individual typically holds any given pose for some time and repeats it several times during the workout which improves both strength and endurance.

- **Yoga improves the posture of seniors**

Yoga is one of the perfect ways to improve one's posture. When you stand straight and tall, shoulders back and relaxed, chin up, chest out, head level, and stomach in, then it is called the perfect posture of an individual.

- **Yoga helps maintain body composition**

Body composition is the percentage of fat that makes up the body, muscles, bones, organs, and other nonfat tissues. Regular yoga exercise decreases the percentage of body fat and oxidative stress and hence it is helpful to reduce the risks of occurrence of various diseases and regulates a healthy lifestyle.

- **Yoga helps mitigate back pain**

Yoga helps in the stretching and strengthening of muscles that generally support the back and spine. It stretches the para-spinal muscles that help bend the spine, while the multifidus muscles and transverse abdomen help balance the vertebrae which helps relieve back pain.

- **Yoga helps you to cope up with stress and anxiety.**

Regular practice of yoga reduces the stress hormones i.e. lowers cortisol levels as well as enhances your mood by increasing the serotonin levels (happy hormones) and induces relaxation as yoga exercises are a combination of body and mind exercises that cultivate the sense of calmness and well-being.

- **Yoga improves cardiorespiratory fitness**

Yoga helps increase your VO2max levels (maximal oxygen uptake which indicates the efficacy of oxygen which can be used by muscles to perform their activity without fatigue) while promoting heart health. Moreover, it also controls high blood pressure and maintains the ideal body weight which also reduces the risk of cardiovascular diseases.

- **Yoga reduces the symptoms of arthritis**

Mind-body exercises such as yoga provide arthritis patients a symptom management strategy to improve physical and mental health. Studies have shown that yoga reduces the symptoms of arthritis and improves physical function.

- **Yoga manages to relieve the symptoms of migraines.**

Research studies show that when an individual adapts to the practice of yoga regularly, then it stimulates the vagus nerve and hence reduces the symptoms of migraine and its intensity/ frequency.

CHAPTER 6: Nutrition Care for Women Over 60 Years

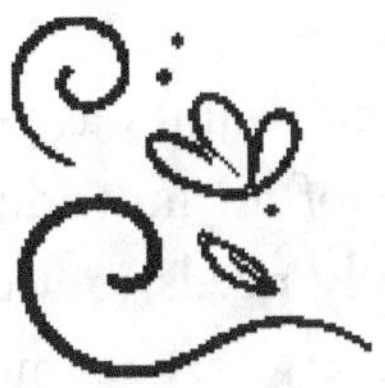

Nutrition care in elderly people is no longer restricted to disease management or medical nutrition therapy but has enhanced to provide a greater reliance on healthy lifestyles and disease prevention. Without a stronger focus on better nutrition and lifestyle modification at all ages, medical expenses will increase as the population ages. Two types of preventive services are included in nutrition. The main focus of primary prevention is on nutrition to promote health and prevent disease. It is equally important to combine healthy eating with physical activity. Secondary prevention requires decreasing the risk of chronic nutrition-related diseases and slowing their progression in order to maintain functionality and quality of life.

General Dietary Guidelines for Women With No Medical History

- **Energy**

The basal metabolic rate (BMR) declines as you age because of changes that occur in the body composition of an individual. The basal metabolic rate is the number of calories your body needs to accomplish its most basic (basal) life-sustaining functions. These energy requirements decline up to 3% after every decade. For energy calculation in elderly women, 2403kcal/day can be suggested. Nutrient-dense foods should be suggested to fulfill caloric needs.

- **Protein**

The minimum protein requirement for women above the age of 60 is 0.80 grams for each pound of body weight. The requirement may vary due to health conditions and absorption. Protein intake helps prevent a person from body muscle mass loss.

- **Carbohydrate**

Carbohydrate requirements for women above the age of 60 are 45%-65% of daily total calories. Mainly carbohydrates are the major source of energy. In older adults, carbohydrate choices should be complex carbs, legumes, and lentils.

Whole grains: cereals, oats, barley, and rice are great choices. Servings of cereals for elderly women are 8-11 servings per day. Fruits and vegetables: 2-4 servings of fruits, 3-5 servings of vegetables, and 21grams of fiber per day are recommended especially for women over 60. Whole grains, fruits, and vegetables are the source of dietary fiber that helps increase the laxation process with older persons.

- **Fats and lipids**

20%-35% of total calories are recommended. Unsaturated fats, oils like omega 6 and 3 are great for older females.

- **Water**

With elderly females, a water intake of at least 1,500ml (1ml =1kcal) is recommended. It helps prevent electrolyte imbalance, constipation, dry mouth, dehydration, fatigue, and blood pressure changes.

- **Mineral and Vitamins**

Vitamin B12: 2.4 mg/day is recommended with older females. Older females at the age of 50 and beyond should eat fortified foods having B12 because with elderly women low intake of B12 causes a decline in gastric juices which could hamper absorption.

Vitamin D: 600-800IU/day is recommended for elderly females. The deficiency risks become higher because both the ability of the skin to expose to sunlight and thus consequently the ability to synthesize vitamin D into an active form by the kidneys declines. So, vitamin D supplements or rich foods are extremely important and recommended.

Folate (folic acid): The recommended value of folate is 400 μg/day. In elderly people, homocysteine levels may decline which is the main risk factor for Alzheimer's disease, atherothrombosis, and Parkinson's disease. Eating grains with folate or taking supplements is a great way to meet your daily demand for folic acid.

Calcium: 1200 mg/day is the dietary requirement of calcium. Unfortunately, only 4% of women at the age of 60 and beyond meet these daily recommendations. The necessary daily intake of calcium increases due to decreased absorption as you age.

Naturally occurring calcium-rich foods and supplements are therefore highly recommended.

Potassium: 4,700 mg/day of potassium is recommended. A potassium-rich diet (bananas) can reduce the effect of sodium causing high blood pressure.

Fruits and vegetables have high amounts of potassium.

Sodium: The recommended amount of sodium is 1,500 mg/day. However, please note that too much sodium causes fluid retention and hypernatremia which trigger the chances of hypertension.

Zinc: Recommended zinc with women at the age of 60 or above is 8 mg/day. A lack of zinc can cause loss of taste, immune function impairment, and delayed wound healing. Therefore, nuts, peanuts, beans, and seeds should be consumed on a regular basis. You could also take a zinc supplement.

Dietary Guidelines for Women Above 60 Having Diabetes

The main focus of medical nutrition therapy (MNT) for women suffering from diabetes is on maintaining and achieving body weight goals although adequate calories can already help maintain weight. Obesity and overweight are the main risk factors of diabetes with elderly women due to lack of physical activity

- **Carbohydrate**

45%-55% is recommended for elderly women suffering from diabetes. Carbohydrates should be chosen wisely. Foods having a low glycemic index and high glycemic load are good at controlling the glycemic effect of the blood, 25g/day of fiber for elderly women is recommended. Fiber helps maintain weight and also helps balance the insulin level. Whole grains, cereals, oats, rice, barley, raw fruits, and vegetables are highly recommended. However, refined flour, bakery products, white flour, fruit juices, and the processed food should be avoided.

- **Fruits and Vegetables**

2-4 fruits servings per day that have a low glycemic index such as apples, berries, strawberries, guava, pear, kiwi, orange, melon are recommended. However, you should avoid high glycemic index fruit such as dates, mangos, and bananas.

3-6 vegetable servings per day should be consumed except for starchy vegetables such as potatoes, turnips, pumpkins.

- **Protein**

The amount of protein that is recommended for diabetic patients is 15-20%.

Protein is the main component of body muscle mass and maintenance of bone health.

- **Fat**

The minimum requirement of fat is 20% and 35% for elderly female diabetic patients. However, the type of fat is more important than the consumption of total fat: monounsaturated fatty acids (MUFAS) such as Omega 6 and polyunsaturated fatty acids (PUFAS) such as Omega 3 are great for your health. So, make sure to make these fats part of your daily diet regime because diabetic patients are more at risk to suffer from cardiovascular diseases (CVDs).

- **Alcohol**

For diabetic patients, drinking alcohol should be done with caution. In fact, the daily intake for women with diabetes should be less than 1 drink =12oz of wine. Light to moderate consumption of alcohol prevents a patient from developing cardiovascular diseases.

Exercise and Physical Activity

Physical activity should be a part of every diabetic's treatment plan. Exercise benefits all diabetics by improving insulin sensitivity, lowering cardiovascular risk factors, controlling weight, and improving overall well-being.

Adults with diabetes should be recommended to engage in at least 150 minutes a week of moderate-intensity aerobic physical exercise (50 percent to 70% of normal heart rate) or at least 90 minutes per week of strength training, vigorous aerobic exercise (more than 70% of maximum heart rate).

Dietary Guidelines for Women Over 60 With Cardiovascular Diseases

- **Weight Management**

In order to lower blood pressure and complication, the body mass index (BMI) should range within 18.5-24.9. Research studies have even shown that overweight and obese individuals with elevated blood pressure who succeed in losing weight by only 3% to 5% imply clinically significant benefits that reduce the need for blood pressure-lowering drugs.

- **Carbohydrate**

The recommended amount of carbohydrates is the same as with healthy women which is 45%-65%. When taking carbohydrates, always make sure to choose complex carbohydrates and to avoid simple carbohydrates in the treatment of cardiovascular diseases.

- **Fruits and Vegetables**

Plant-based dietary habits have been linked to lower systolic blood pressure (SBP) in clinical trials. SBP reductions of 5-6 on average have been recorded. The Dietary Approaches to Stop Hypertension (DASH) have proven that a dietary pattern promoting fruits, vegetables, low-fat products, whole grains, lean meats, and nuts reduce significantly blood pressure. Eat 5 to 10 servings of fruits and vegetables per day for a significant reduction in CVD.

- **Protein**

The protein requirement of a diabetic patient is 0.8g per kg of body weight. Medium or less fat protein is a great option for patients suffering from CVD.

- **Lipid**

Current dietary lipid composition guidelines are recommended to aid in weight loss and reduce the chances of CVD. Saturated and trans fats should be avoided. Their consumption may cause hyperlipidemia and atherosclerosis. Intake of omega 3 has great benefits for patients suffering from CVDs.

- **Alcohol**

Alcohol intake should be limited to not more than one drink for women with diabetic issues. Excessive consumption of alcohol causes hypertension, hyperlipidemia, and other cardiovascular diseases.

- **Sodium**

Less than 2300mg of sodium is recommended. Due to The Dietary Approaches to Stop Hypertension (DASH), 1600mg/day of sodium consumption is recommended. Please note that foods having high sodium cause hypertension along with its complications.

- **Potassium**

1,900mg to 4,700 mg of potassium helps lower the risk of hypertension. Less consumption of sodium and high consumption of potassium helps decrease the risk of a stroke. A diet that is too low in potassium causes sodium-sensitive hypertension.

- **Magnesium**

Due to The Dietary Approaches to Stop Hypertension, a diet should contain magnesium-rich food to control or prevent hypertension. The daily recommendation of magnesium for women over 60 is 320-370mg/day.

- **Calcium and Vitamin D**

1,200mg/day of Calcium is recommended. Cross-sectional studies show that deficiency of vitamin D and calcium are significantly related to high blood pressure.

Exercise and Physical Activity

Less active people are more subject to suffer from CVD. Exercise plays an important role in the prevention and control of hypertension. Light to moderate intensity of 30 to 40 minutes of physical activity is recommended. It also helps lower blood pressure.

Dietary Guidelines for Osteoporosis

- **Energy**

For optimum bone health, body mass index (BMI) should range within 18.5-24.9. Being underweight or overweight affects bone health and becomes the underlying cause of osteopenia and osteoporosis.

- **Protein and Calcium**

Adequate calcium and adequate protein intake both are directly proportional to bone health. The recommendation of calcium is 1,200mg per day for elderly females.

- **Vitamin D**

800-1000 units/day of vitamin D is recommended for females above 60 having osteoporosis in order to prevent fractures. You can take supplements of vitamin D to make sure you meet your daily intake.

- **Vitamin K**

For bone health, vitamin K is an essential micronutrient. The Recommended Dietary Allowance (RDA) of vitamin K is 1mcg per kg of body weight. Dark green leafy vegetables are one of the major sources of vitamin K. In many cases, older people have inadequate intake of vitamin K due to very low consumption of green vegetables. Vitamin K consumption is also very important with older people taking medication for blood-thinning or anticlotting.

- **Dietary habits**

A balanced diet of low-fat, fruit, whole grains, and vegetables that include adequate content of calcium and vitamin D is recommended by the National Osteoporosis Foundation. Maintaining weight and intake of a low sodium diet also helps support bone health.

Exercise and Physical Activity

Exercises that require a lot of force on potentially weakened tissue, such as sit-ups or bending, are not recommended for people who have osteoporosis. Walking regularly and swimming are therefore more recommended for older people.

Dietary Guidelines for Chronic Kidney Diseases

- **Energy**

Energy requirements depend upon the patient condition and comorbidities along with the disease.

- **Protein**

Protein requirements vary from person to person with the severity of the disease. The ideal protein intake should be 0.5-0.8g per kg of body weight for a non-dialysis patient. However, for patients receiving dialysis, it should be 1-2g per kg of body weight.

- **Fluid and sodium**

An Intake of fluid and sodium of 20-40 mEq/day depending on urine output, edema, and serum sodium level is recommended. Excessive fluid and sodium may cause water retention in renal patients.

- **Potassium**

Excretion and control of potassium are mostly done by the kidneys. In renal disease, kidneys are not able to perform their function properly. As a result, potassium overloading may occur. Intake of potassium may vary between 30-50 mEq/day according to patient serum potassium levels depending on urine output, and edema.

- **Phosphorus**

The level of serum phosphorus increases with a decrease in renal function. Hyperphosphatemia causes hyperthyroidism and bone diseases. Restriction of phosphorus or intake of phosphate binder is a great way to treat renal diseases.

- **Lipids**

Low-fat diets are encouraged in MNT (medical nutrition therapy) for renal disease. Intake of a high-fat diet causes the risk of hyperlipidemia and cardiovascular disease. Consumption of monounsaturated fatty acids (MUFAS) and polyunsaturated fatty acids (PUFAS) in combination with adequate protein helps in reducing the chances of low-density cholesterol.

Diet sample chart for women above the age of 60

Timings	Diet
Breakfast	1 cup oatmeal with organic coconut milk with fruits (banana, blueberries, figs) and 1 tsp honey.
Snacks	1 cup apple quinoa salad or 2 cucumbers of medium size and fruit of your choice
Lunch	1 cup cooked whole-wheat (pasta or spaghetti) with ½ cup cooked vegetables (cabbage, carrots, bell peppers properly boiled or shredded)
Snacks	1 cup raw fruits or 1 cup beetroot juice
Dinner	Spinach soup with 1 small whole-grain bread. Or 1 cup rice bran and 1 cup of veggies.

CHAPTER 7: Meditation

Meditation is a natural exercise that everyone can do to relieve tension, improve calmness and clarity, and encourage happiness. Learning to meditate is easy, and the benefits can be noticed quickly. Meditation is a method of training focus and perception, as well as achieving a mentally clear and emotionally relaxed, and stable state. This is achieved by strategies such as mindfulness or focusing the mind on a specific object, thinking, or behavior. Meditation has been shown to relieve stress, anxiety, depression, and pain. It also helps improve peace, awareness, self-concept, and overall well-being. Paying attention to the breath, a concept or feeling such as mett (loving-kindness) or a mantra (such as in transcendental meditation), and single point meditation are examples of focused approaches.

The Basics

We may be more concerned with our physical well-being as we get older, but that does not mean we should neglect our mental health. There are several physical and psychological advantages of mindful meditation. People have been meditating since 5,000 BC, so it's nothing new. Setting aside time for formal meditation is crucial for developing a routine and becoming relaxed with the activity. Even a few minutes a day can have a significant impact on your life. Some people are irritated by the fact that it takes time out of their day. However, that's not the case at all. It is much more investing in the day ahead. And like anything else in life you need to practice meditation in order to become good at it. It's a technique for bringing yourself back into balance during stressful circumstances. When we stop meditating, however, we do not stop being conscious. While self-meditation is an important part of a complete practice, having the steady guidance of an experienced instructor can be extremely beneficial, particularly as you progress. Our minds wander easily, and a teacher's straightforward guide will help us return to focusing.

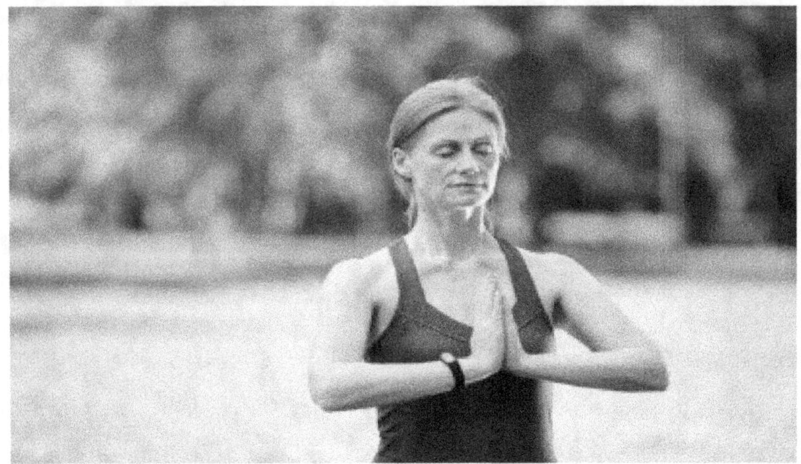

It's almost impossible to even spend a short while meditating without being distracted by ringing smartphones, flickering computer screens, and up-to-the-second breaking news updates in today's always-on culture. This is very detrimental to older women's fitness and health. So, in order to meditate, you need to switch off any distraction sources before. Consider meditation if you're looking for a way to avoid the relentless barrage of anxiety, frustration, resentment, self-doubt, restlessness, and inner self-talk caused by daily stresses. It will help you manage your tension, increase your productivity, and provide you with a more relaxed and healthier body.

Benefits of Meditation

- **Lowers Stress, Regulates Hormones, and Controls Menopause Symptoms**

Meditation's primary goal is to calm the mind, relax the body and promote a higher degree of consciousness and wisdom in order to get the body, mind, and spirit into balance. The indirect result is a decrease in tension. We all know that stress causes a variety of health issues, including high blood pressure, heart disease, and depression. Pressure, muscle tightness, and back and neck spasms are all symptoms of stress, and they can make daily life difficult. Meditation is a technique for calming the mind and soothing the soul, allowing you to see things in a calmer light and with more serenity rather than frantic anxiety.

- **Meditation counteracts the negative effects of stress hormones on our bodies and minds.**

Meditators are better able to deal with acute emotional distress and daily stressors because they can instinctively stabilize these emotions. Controlled breathing will eventually stimulate your body's hormone-balancing response.

- **Increases Productivity**

One of life's greatest and most rewarding simple pleasures is completing all of the tasks you set out to do in a day. It's amazing how stress fades away and pleasure can be felt in everyday activities when you can focus unwaveringly on your goals, free of distractions and the stress of meeting other people's needs. Milestones provide us with a feeling of pride and pleasure. If you find yourself accomplishing less than you like, feeling exhausted, and jumping from one task to the next, meditation may be able to help you approach tasks calmly and with a clearer focus. In order to sharpen your concentration and relax flustered anxiety and frayed nerves, start your day with light exercise as little as 12 minutes of meditation. According to the American Psychological Association, "Mindful Meditation" improves memory, calms and stabilizes emotions, and allows the mind to solve problems more effectively.

- **Reduces Pain Pill Consumption**

According to Prevention magazine, meditation can alleviate discomfort and, as a result, the amount of pain medication needed to keep our aging bodies comfortable. Pain sensation originates in the nerve centers of our brains, just above the brainstem, which is maybe more important. Zen meditation, which emphasizes posture and breathing, literally thickens this area of the brain.

Meditation's benefits are almost limitless when paired with a variety of allopathic and modern medical treatments. Pressure relief, brain tissue regeneration, and hormone balancing properties have far-reaching effects.

How Can Mindful Meditation Benefit Seniors?

For older adults, mindful meditation has many possible physical and psychological benefits, including improved concentration, increased calmness, reduced tension, and improved sleep. Mindfulness and meditation have been shown in studies to alleviate stress and pain while also improving mental well-being. It can also assist adults in dealing with the struggles of growing older. Meditation has been linked to improved short-term and long-term memory. According to research studies, it can also delay the development of Alzheimer's disease. Meditation seems to be able to counteract age-related cognitive loss, according to preliminary evidence. It not only activates the "feel-good" prefrontal cortex, but it can also alter the brain's structure to increase concentration, imagination, and cognitive function.

How to do Mindful Meditation?

Make time and room for yourself. Start small. While you want to work up to 20 minutes a day, this can be difficult to achieve at first. You can practice mindful meditation at any time and in any location, even if you have mobility or agility issues.

Begin by sitting or lying down in a comfortable place. Deep diaphragmatic breaths are recommended. Concentrate on inhaling and exhaling and pay attention to all other physical stimuli the body is expressing. Check the stance when you're lying down or standing.

Don't miss out!

Visit the website below and you can sign up to receive emails whenever Dr. Robertino Bedenian publishes a new book. There's no charge and no obligation.

https://books2read.com/r/B-A-YQGQ-DPWPB

BOOKS 2 READ

Connecting independent readers to independent writers.

Also by Dr. Robertino Bedenian

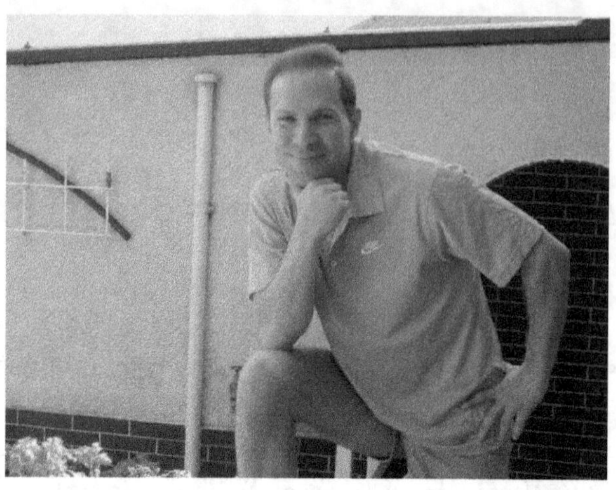

About the Author

Dr. Robertino Bedenian is a qualified fitness instructor accredited by the German Olympic Committee, a health and nutrition expert, and the author of several books on diet, health, and fitness!

For more than twenty years he has been a fitness coach at the sports university teaching aerobics, back gymnastics, stretching, high-intensity interval training (HIIT), power gymnastics, and athletic sports.

On his website, he has published more than 300 articles about the vegan lifestyle covering diet and health recommendations, detoxication programs, fitness guidelines, and disease-related topics. He is part of a family with an orthopedic surgeon, a physical therapist, an osteopath, and an alternative practitioner.

He is also the founder of the brand "**Going Vegan**" selling high-quality supplements for optimal health.

You are more than welcome to check his website for more details: https://goingveganhealthbenefits.com.

His brand has been awarded continuously with 5-star feedback by customers for its outstanding product quality.

Dr. Bedenian is also the founder of the book company "**Book Summary Publishing**" publishing summaries and workbooks of Amazon #1 bestselling non-fiction books.

If you want to learn more about the summaries and workbooks that he has published so far, please visit his website:

www.ingramcontent.com/pod-product-compliance
Lightning Source LLC
Chambersburg PA
CBHW070549160726

48003CB00005B/1964